ROUND EYES

An American Nurse in Vietnam

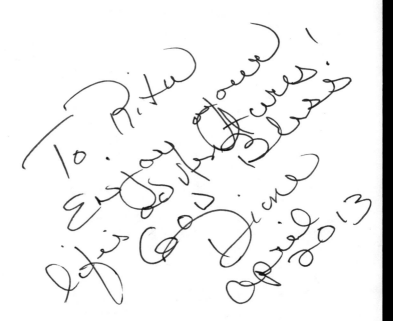

ROUND EYES

An American Nurse in Vietnam

Diane Klutz

TRI-STAR BOOKS
***

Library of Congress Control Number: 2012931434
ISBN: 978-1-889987-11-8

Cover and book designer: James Retherford/Hot Digital Dog Design. Typography: *text* Melior; *titles* Futura.

Copy editor: Robert Juran.

Printed in USA.

First Printing.

CREDITS

Front cover inset photo: helicopter medevac (VA042547), James Evans Collection, August 1970, The Vietnam Center and Archive, Texas Tech University. *Front and back cover snapshots:* the author's personal collection.

Elizabeth Norman, *Women at War: The Story of Fifty Military Nurses Who Served in Vietnam* (Philadelphia: University of Pennsylvania Press, 1990). Reproduced with the permission of the author.

Florence Nightingale, *Notes on Nursing: What It Is, and What It Is Not* (New York: D. Appleton, 1860).

Florence Nightingale, *Florence Nightingale to Her Nurses: A Selection From Miss Nightingale's Addresses to Proba-tioners and Nurses of the Nightingale School, St. Thomas' Hospital* (London: Macmillan, 1914).

Helen Wells, *Cherry Ames, Army Nurse* (New York: Grosset & Dunlap, 1944). Reproduced with the permission of Springer Publishing Company, LLC.

TRI-STAR BOOKS

***

CONTENTS

DEDICATION

This story is dedicated
to all the military nurses
who volunteered to care
for the physically and
mentally wounded soldiers,
the dying soldiers,
and the civilians
in South Vietnam.

It wasn't easy,
and it still may not be,
but you did it anyway.

ACKNOWLEDGEMENTS

A very special "thank you" goes to Capt. Robert Schuster, USN Ret., who is my uncle and my publisher. Without his guidance, this book would not have made it off my computer screen. The easy part was writing the manuscript; the hard part was figuring out what to do once it was written. Uncle Bob made that happen.

Appreciation also goes to copy editor Robert Juran who took time from his busy schedule to review my manuscript, not once but twice. His input was invaluable.

I want to acknowledge my friends, Cindy, Merry, and Linda Kay, who repeatedly said, "You need to write a book." Okay, girlfriends, you can let up now.

Thank you to my daughter Shannon who not only provided recommendations for chapter placement but also kept reminding me of stories that I forgot to include.

And a great big "thank you" to Stephen, my husband, who supported me through this process and wisely did not read the manuscript until I finished. Thank you, Sweetie, for your patience.

Nursing had always been Cherry's dream. She knew it was the finest way a girl could serve people, and Cherry loved people and wanted to help them. Nursing was the way to put her idealism into practice.

— Helen Wells, *Cherry Ames, Army Nurse*, p. 13

PROLOGUE

A Little Background First

Before I begin my story, I need to set the stage by giving you a sense of knowing me: who I was and how that may have led me to the Vietnam War.

My life began in a rural community of about 200 people in southwestern Pennsylvania, close to the border of West Virginia. A fort established in the early 1700s, called Fort Taylor, formed the basis and hence the name for the town — Taylorstown.

Patriotism flowed through Taylorstown's blood in proportions equal to that of red or white blood cells. My family and I shared the commonality of patriotism so evident in the community. I'm proud to say that there has been at least one member of my family in every war since the forming of the colonies: from the French and Indian War through the current wars in Iraq and Afghanistan.

The first five years of my elementary education were in a four- room schoolhouse, and the sixth grade was in a single-room schoolhouse. There was no indoor plumbing in our schools, but at least there were separate outhouses for girls and boys — three-holers at that. My grandmother only had a one-holer. Anyway, by the time I reached junior high a new school was built, with indoor plumbing and everything.

I graduated from high school in June 1966, and two months later I started nurse's training in a girls-only school in a hospital north of Pittsburgh. I was seventeen, and I had never been away from home before. And I was a little naïve since there were three boys and just one girl (me) in our family. Actually, I was so naïve that I thought feminine napkins were table napkins used exclusively by ladies. It was after my girlfriend and I got caught by a teacher, while carrying a box of these "napkins" from the ladies bathroom to the cafeteria, that I learned what they were actually used for — I was so embarrassed.

In nursing school, I lived in the dorm with the other nursing students. In fact, everyone lived in the dorm married or not, children or not. This was usually not an issue, because marriage was forbidden until the student was close to graduation. However, a few girls came into the program married, and one of my classmates was divorced, with custody of her two children. But no matter what the circumstances were, without exception, everyone stayed in the dorm.

The dorm was connected like an umbilical cord to the hospital and much like living in a womb — very protected and structured. We ate, slept, studied, and did nearly everything according to set rules. While freshmen, we were allowed out of the building for free time only from 6 to 8 p.m., Monday through Thursday. On Friday and Saturday we could stay out until 10 p.m. Juniors were permitted to stay out to 9 p.m. on weekdays and seniors till 10. Everyone had to be back in the dorm by 8 p.m. on Sundays. All classes were held in the basement of the dorm, and a few were in the hospital area. Meals were in the student cafeteria, also located in the basement. Except when we had specialty training rotations, we incubated and grew into nurses within the uterus of the hospital.

After thirty six straight months of confinement, the womb opened and I graduated. It was August 1969 and I was twenty years old. I worked in a local hospital for four months after graduation. The first week of January 1970 I was commissioned into active duty as a second lieutenant in the United States Army Nurse Corps. The following week Mom and Dad drove me to the airport in Pittsburgh, and even though it was snowing, they stood outside, watching as I climbed the steps, and after a final wave I disappeared into the plane.

I wish to salute you young women who are about to become Army nurses! You will take the first steps today.

> — Lieutenant Colonel Wylie addressing the new recruits. Helen Wells, *Cherry Ames, Army Nurse*, p. 56

Basic Training

I felt like Amelia Earhart heading across the Atlantic as I joined the plane full of newly commissioned Army nurses heading for basic training at Fort Sam Houston in San Antonio, Texas. Most of us had never left Pennsylvania, yet alone visited Texas, and we were so excited to be going to the home of the Alamo.

Fort Sam Houston, Fort Sam for short, was the training site for all Army medical personnel. Nurses, doctors, dentists, physical therapists, and all other officers in an Army medical field had to successfully complete the six-week basic training course at Fort Sam.

It was January 1970, and by the time we arrived on post the sun had long ago settled into the western sky. Most of the rooms in the nurses' dorm were already assigned, so many of us from the Pittsburgh area were housed in the married officers' dorm. These quarters additionally housed the male nurses along with married nurse couples, physicians, and dentists. Even though men and women didn't have to share bathroom facilities, it still seemed strange to see men in the hall, especially in their underwear.

I guess the Army did its best to prepare us nurses for military service. We had day-long lectures about weapons of all makes and sizes, tactical maneuvers, military protocol, war strategy, and other stuff too boring to remember. And we marched — in heels, combat boots, dress uniforms, and pants.

We participated in field exercises, which were actually fun. We experienced the fine culinary delight of C-rations and food served in a mess tent. We removed shrapnel and debrided wounds on goats, set up and took down medical tents, and suffered through tear gas instruction, while wearing full combat gear.

We were even set loose in the middle of the wilderness at Camp Bullis with a navigation map and a compass. Presumably, we were to find our way back to camp, but our group got lost. Fortunately there were warrant officers in helicopters chomping at the bit to rescue any stray nurses, so it wasn't long before help arrived.

What the Army did not prepare us for were the men. Willing and able officers were everywhere, just waiting for an opportunity to take out a new recruit. And there was always a band playing at either the senior officers' clubs or junior officers' clubs. Because several of the clubs stayed open until the wee hours of the morning, and there was no curfew, I occasionally had two or three dates in one night. Shamefully, a few times I got back to my room just in time to wash, fix hair and makeup, change into my uniform, and run to formation.

"I now am," she reminded herself, remembering her oath of office, *"by act of Congress, an officer and a Lady."*

— Helen Wells, *Cherry Ames, Army Nurse*, p. 56

The Reflecting Pool

I suppose the lack of sleep accounted for my inability to absorb much during class time, especially when the finer points of the disciplined military life were discussed. In fact, I pretty much ignored the whole thing, because I was focused on another topic: having fun.

I also had, and still have, a major character flaw: accepting authority. I never cultivated this attitude; it just happened. Hearing "just because" to my "why" questions never sat well with me. In addition, trouble seemed to hang around me like a cloud. I certainly did not go looking for it, but it was there nonetheless and usually the outcome of these encounters ended very close to disaster.

One of these encounters with trouble occurred several months after graduating from basic training and Fort Sam Houston. I was assigned to Walter Reed Medical Center in Washington, D.C. Another nurse in my basic training class, named Cindy, was given the same duty assignment, and because Walter Reed did not have on-post housing, we decided to share an apartment together.

Cindy and I were off duty on a particularly beautiful spring Saturday afternoon. The year was 1970, and a celebration was planned by the D.C. Parks Department to commemorate Congress' recent reversal of the kite-flying law. Up to that point, kite flying was restricted near the National Mall, because no building or other type of structure could be higher than the Washington Monument, including kites. I guess it was some special law written long before airplanes and such were invented.

The weatherman promised a magnificent day: clear skies and sun. Kites were provided by the Parks Department, and throngs of enthusiasts, Cindy and I included, descended on the monument grounds. As if on cue, no sooner did the kites take flight than the sky burst forth with rain, lightning, thunder, and hail. Mad dashes were made to shelters, cars, pavilions, and whatever else was handy. Thankfully, as suddenly as the storm started, it stopped, and the sun exploded from behind the storm clouds.

Those of you who were familiar with the National Mall area of the 1970s may remember that there were many grass-covered knolls, especially surrounding the amphitheater. A few of the knolls' banks were quite steep and provided inclined seating to watch outdoor performances. I once watched Dionne Warwick perform in this amphitheater.

Anyway, after the downpour, the grass on the bank became slippery, proving irresistible to many of the festival participants. Like otters, the soaking mass of people who were previously flying kites began sliding down the embankment, turning the grass carpet into a giant mudslide.

Throngs of people, mostly in their twenties, joined in the frolicking on the muddy banks of the mall. Cindy and I couldn't resist having at least one slide, but because there were so many packed-in people, the ride wasn't fast or long. But it sure was muddy.

Perfect recollections are now lost to time, but not long after the grassy banks turned into a thick chocolate-like slide, a single voice was heard. "Let's go to the Reflecting Pool to wash off this mud," said the unknown male, and like sheep to the slaughter the mud-covered group turned and followed this unknown and unseen leader. Thinking that this was a "groovy" plan, I coaxed Cindy into also going to the pool. We sat on the short wall encompassing the pool and dangled our feet while others splashed and cavorted in the shallow water. Cindy remarked at one point that this was probably illegal, but because we weren't positive, we kept our perch on the wall splashing our feet.

The sun was shining, people were laughing, and music was blaring. There were even rainbows in the sky. Everything seemed right in the world ... when without warning a man wearing Army-surplus combat fatigues and a plethora of peace signs started shouting anti-war rhetoric via a bullhorn. The man's voice sounded very much like the unknown leader to the pool's voice — probably not a coincidence.

While others joined the newly created protest, Cindy and I just stared at the spectacle, and at each other. One moment we were flying kites and the next we were smack dab in the middle of an anti-war rally. And we were officers in the United States Army. Court martial was the only thought running through my mind as Cindy yanked me out of the water. This was really going to be bad.

Then bad became worse. Buses rolled to a stop on an access street on the small hill above the Reflecting Pool. Police in riot gear emerged, forming a perimeter line around the now-quiet crowd in the pool. Of course, the bullhorn-toting protester did not stop his ranting against the president and the government, but Cindy and I were too scared to pay attention.

Like skilled Green Berets, we assumed the belly-crawl position and elbowed our way toward the riot police. Then, spotting a break in the line, we ran as fast as we could away from the commotion. Tear gas formed around us like a cloud stinging our eyes. Coughing and sputtering, we made it to our car and raced home.

The national news that evening featured the protest, including the bullhorn leader and the Reflective Pool bath-ers. Thankfully, neither Cindy's face nor mine stared back as we nervously watched the television screen. "Safe," we sighed as the broadcast ended without MPs knocking at our door.

However, our reprieve wasn't as long as desired, for only a few months later we received our personal "Welcome to Vietnam" letter.

*The plane was heading for the jungles —
perhaps for the smoky, deafening air of
battle. Cherry did not know what new life
she would find there, what new challenge
she would face. But whatever it was, she
was ready for it!*

— Helen Wells, *Cherry Ames, Army Nurse*, p. 214

ONE

The Beginning

I stepped out of the Tiger Airlines plane into the broiler-oven night of Southeast Asia. It was mid-November 1970, and the air was solid with humidity — so much that I couldn't take a breath. Or maybe it was the sight of soldiers armed with machine guns surrounding the plane that smothered all my respiratory effort. And the soldiers looked so young.

I had just celebrated my twenty-second birthday, but I looked at least a decade older than these boys.

We were told during basic training that most of us would be sent to Vietnam within the year, so my being there should not have surprised me. I guess I just never thought it could really happen.

Like a worm tunneling its way through clay, the reality of the situation ebbed into my consciousness. My mind swirled with an overwhelming sense of dread mixed with the excitement of adventure. My roommate Cindy and another Army nurse, Major Marilyn Watson, were also on this flight, but they had already left the plane. My feet felt nailed in place, but I forced them down the steps to catch up with the other two. As we passed between the gauntlets of armed soldiers lining the tarmac, I wondered what the future would hold and how I ever got myself into this mess.

I have to admit that I had a bit of longing for adventure. I watched *MASH* (the movie) at least three times. I had all the nurses' parts memorized. As a young teenager, I had read most of the *Cherry Ames* novels, including *Student Nurse*, *Senior Nurse*, *Army Nurse*, *Chief Nurse*, *Flight Nurse*, and *Veteran's Nurse*. I dreamed of being Tammy in *Tammy and the Doctor*. I pictured myself as a modern-day Florence Nightingale fighting to save soldiers' lives, side by side in the mud with fellow nurses and doctors. And now I was here; it would be my time of glory.

Lost in my assortment of thoughts, I didn't notice that Cindy and Major Watson were no longer close by. I finally found them; they were loading themselves and their duffel bags onto a bus. I ran to grab my duffel bag, but it was nowhere to be found. I searched frantically, but still no duffel bag. I panicked. After twenty-four solid hours in the same underwear and travel uniform, I was in dire need of a change. Then my name seared the silence as it was blared over the airport loudspeakers: I was to board the bus immediately, and so I did, minus my duffel bag.

Now for those who have never experienced the joy of travel, military style, there were certain essentials of deployment packing for Vietnam.

The first was the foot locker. This held your year's worth of necessities: hair curlers, hair dryer, hair color, casual clothes, socks, snacks, toiletries, personal ladies' items, and underwear.

Because your foot locker might take one to two months to find you, a duffel bag was next. This held intermediate necessities: hair curlers, makeup, hair color, shampoo and conditioners, toiletries, and monthly female necessities.

The third was a small carry-on tote bag, which held the real necessities: makeup, toiletries, a few female necessities, and at least one change of underwear. However, because I was a true believer in Merle Norman, my tote was abundant with lipstick, makeup base, powder, eyeliner, eye shadow, and mascara. I did manage to pack deodorant, but I forgot the underwear.

Ordinarily this would not be a problem. In the real world, I would simply go to the closest K-Mart or Montgomery Ward's store and purchase new undergarments. But I wasn't in the real world; I was in Vietnam.

My mother's words loomed in my head: "Always wear clean underwear in case you're in an accident. You don't want doctors and nurses seeing you in dirty under-

wear." It was like a hex: wearing dirty under-wear in pub-
lic doomed the offender to an emergency-room visit. The
fact that I was a registered nurse with emergency training
and up to that point had never once withheld treatment
for a patient because of dirty underwear did not alter my
foreboding thoughts.

I bet Florence Nightingale or Cherry Ames never
forgot to pack spare underwear. I was fast becoming a fail-
ure to the nursing profession.

TWO

Disillusioned

Epiphany moments happen along one's life journey, and I soon realized this night was one for me. As the bus lumbered through a village not far from the airport, emotions twirled in my being like a spinning top. First was fear — I was scared to death. There were soldiers with guns in and on top of the bus. It was the middle of the night, yet the dusty streets were jammed with soldiers in jeeps, people on bikes, and villagers walking around hawking their wares.

This wasn't right. Where were the smiling mamasans with long dresses wearing woven coned hats? Why weren't these people happy to see us, their American liberators? Where was the throng of cheering, flower-pelting grateful people like those who cheered the Americans when they liberated France in World War II? All I saw was filth, sad faces, sewage in the streets, hovels crowded with children and adults, and more filth. I was confused and disgusted.

The truth of the situation slowly sank in. They had lied. The United States government had lied, my teachers had lied, the Army had lied, and God knows who else was in on the lie. I had believed in a cause that wasn't there. I felt angry, betrayed, and not very patriotic at that point.

As tears welled in my eyes, I remarked to Cindy, "This is so sad. No one here gives a rat's ass if they are communist, socialist, or good old capitalists. They are just trying to exist, moment to moment."

Cindy simply nodded in agreement, but as the bus crawled through the city streets she whispered, "Please try to keep your thoughts to yourself. We don't want to get in trouble."

I accepted her sage advice, but silently I brooded, "How could we be doing this to these people? How did this happen?" There wasn't an answer that justified what I saw outside the bus, and deep in my soul I knew I would always remember.

THREE

In-Processing

My anger gave way to nervous anticipation as the bus pulled through the guarded gate at the post where we would be "in-country processed." I had not a clue where I was, where I would be stationed, or whether Cindy and I would be stationed together. Thoughts of being sent to an outpost alone, along with visions of Hot Lips, Hawkeye, and Radar, continued as I walked though what was left of the night to go to the female sleeping quarters.

Actually, sleeping quarters was not the term that came to mind as I stepped into the tent-like structure. There was a ceiling fan but it didn't work. There were sheets on the cots, but I think the last time they were washed was when the French fought for control of Vietnam a generation earlier. A bare bulb, hanging from a ceiling cord, cast a dim light around the room, attracting mosquitoes seemingly as big as horses. Turning off the light was impossible, because the bulb chain was too high to reach.

Batting at the behemoth bloodsuckers, Cindy and I began the search for mosquito nets, or at least repellent. Suddenly a loud deep booming sound reverberated through the building. This was followed shortly by another boom. Cindy, I, and several other newby nurses raced outside to see what was happening. We found a young munchkin-like soldier guarding our quarters. "That's only perimeter mortar fire; outgoing, not incoming," he patiently explained as we all started talking at once. "And it will continue all night, every night."

Great! Pretending reassurance, we scurried back to our mosquito-infested room. I huddled under the vintage sheets and finally drifted off to sleep amid the chainsaw buzzing of the insects and the booming of mortar rounds.

The sun was barely peeking over the trees surrounding the compound when I awoke with the comforting thought that I had survived my first night in Vietnam. Following a breakfast of powdered eggs and acid coffee, Cindy and I, along with the other new nurses, began in-country processing. This was much the same as in any other part of the military: filling out forms, standing in long lines, and filling out more forms.

My last queuing of the day was getting outfitted for jungle fatigues, boots, and other essentials. My brain shifted back to my missing underwear. Surely Army supply people would have underwear. After all, the Army knew women were in South Vietnam as well as men, didn't they? I mean, they sent us here.

My arms were soon full of fatigues, socks, and undershirts (all in lovely green), but no women's underpants. Piled on top of this were my flak jacket, helmet, poncho, boonie hat, and boots. Still no lady's underwear.

With trepidation I approached the clerk, a man, at the end of the line. I discreetly asked where I might find ladies' underpants. He seemed not to hear my request. I repeated the question, a little louder. Feigning a hearing disability, he asked me to repeat my request. I did, and he actually started laughing at me, an officer. What happened to his discipline, his discretion?

"Try the PX [Army language for Post Exchange]. They might have panties," shouted the helpful, deaf clerk. I was as mortified as the day I walked down the main street of my home town, wearing white shorts and not knowing I had started my menstrual period.

Well, I hadn't started my period and I wasn't wearing white shorts, but I was just as embarrassed. Attempting to explain to the Vietnamese ladies working at the PX what I needed was no easy task, either. I knew no Vietnamese and they knew no ladies' underwear language, so after sign language and male assistance, I ended up with three pair of men's skivvies. My mother was never convinced that my lack of female underpants was due to Army neglect.

It was a poster, and on it was a boy in khaki who looked like her own brother Charlie. His rifle was stuck upright into the earth; he was kneeling and clinging to the rifle with both hands, his head drooping.

— Helen Wells, *Cherry Ames, Army Nurse,* p. 16

FOUR

Major "Uncle" Frank

Cindy and I finally received our duty station orders: both of us, along with Major Watson, were going to the Sixty Seventh Evacuation Hospital (67th EVAC for short) in Qui Nhon. We were a little concerned to learn the hospital was in I Corps, which meant it was in the northern part of South Vietnam. The good news was that it was south of Da Nang and adjacent to the South China Sea, with beautiful white beaches and turquoise water. We figured it could be a lot worse.

I had something extremely important to do before I left for the 67th. My little brother Jay was still in Vietnam, as far as I knew. He had been in the country since December 1969 and was scheduled to go home soon. My attempts to locate him before I left the States were not successful, but I was determined to see him. Jay was a chaplain's assistant, so my plan was to resume the search at the post chaplain's building.

An enlisted man was working the communications board at the chapel, and after I finished my story he set to work to find my brother. Less than twenty four hours later, I heard my name being called over the loudspeaker to report to the captain's office. I walked in and noticed the hulking form of a major waiting for me. Before I could question his identity, Jay burst in the door. We stared at each other in disbelief: Jay because he didn't know I was coming to Vietnam, and I because Jay was actually here, all nineteen years of him, in person. I was so excited that I didn't know whether to laugh or cry, so I did both.

Before either of us had a chance to talk, the massive major turned to the Officer of the Day, who was in charge. In a booming voice he introduced himself as Major Frank Smith, chaplain for such-and-such division. And, by the way, he added with emphasis, he was our uncle.

I was dumbfounded. As far as I knew, we had no ministers, preachers, or priests in our family. On top of that, I had never seen this man in my life, but there he stood, requesting a pass for me to leave the camp so we could go to dinner. Jay paled and looked like he was going to throw up. Later he told me that he and the major were not exactly on friendly terms.

Anyway, the request quickly progressed to a demand, as Major "Uncle" Frank insisted that I be allowed to leave. The captain finally relented, after being barraged by the major's litany of family responsibility and duty. I felt like Dorothy in the Land of Oz. I was in South Vietnam, in the middle of a war, with my brother whom I hadn't seen in over a year, and going out to dinner with my newfound preacher uncle.

Trust me, I was and still am a sinner as much as the next girl — or should I say lieutenant. I've told my little fibs to get out of difficult situations, followed by groveling to God to forgive me in accord with my deep remorse and promise to behave forever. However, I was a mere toddler in the fibbing department in comparison to Major "Uncle" Frank as he fabricated family stories to the captain.

Then, to make matters worse, Jay grabbed Major Frank, gave this bear of a man a big hug, and exclaimed loudly, "Uncle Frank, you are the best! Mom is going to be so happy."

Major "Uncle" Frank glared at Jay, grabbed him and me, and out the door we went. Jay hardly made it into the jeep's back seat when Major Frank gunned the engine and sped out the gate. I guess he thought it would be best if we were already gone, in case the captain discovered the truth about our family ties.

That night and even the less turbulent nights that followed tested Cherry's idealism and her worthiness to be an Army nurse to the upmost.

— Helen Wells, *Cherry Ames, Army Nurse*, p. 193

FIVE

The Reality of War

P eople are trained much the same as animals in response to fear stimuli. During the 1950s and early '60s we hunkered under our desks at school during air raid drills. Fire drills caused even the most unruly student to file silently out of a building. Whatever instinct caused us to react as kids continued in Vietnam.

Any loud boom resulted in wrapping of arms around the head and falling to the ground. Occasionally this was just as hazardous as bullets. I heard stories of several soldiers who received Purple Hearts not from direct wounds but as a result of hitting their heads on the floor or bed rails following a loud explosion. It didn't seem to matter whether the mortar rounds were incoming or outgoing.

To illustrate, one night at about 0200 hours (2 a.m. civilian time), Cindy and another nurse were in the process of moving a soldier from the operating room to recovery. This young man, fresh from the boonies, had undergone emergency surgery for appendicitis at the 67th EVAC. He was sleeping the sleep of the anesthetized on a gurney when an incoming mortar hit the ammo dump near the hospital. The ensuing explosion rocked everything within a three-mile radius, including our hospital.

Instinctively, Cindy and the other nurse wrapped their arms over their heads, closed their eyes, and ducked. Moments later, while rising from their floor-hugging position, they saw that their patient was no longer on the gurney. Looking underneath it, they found him on the floor, holding his IV bottle in his hand. "If you think I was going to wait for you two to save me, you have another thought coming." With that, he fell back to sleep.

While Cindy was rolling her patient out of surgery, I was working on the Medical Ward. A newly arrived physician from near Saigon was regaling one of the corpsmen with his military combat expertise when the explosion hit. Shards of glass from the taped windows showered down on the patients, as many scrambled under their cots. Following a second explosion, I yelled for the physician to help the corpsmen cover the immobile patients with mattresses, but he did not respond. One of the patients started having a seizure, so I grabbed a mattress off an empty cot and threw myself and the mattress on top of him.

Thankfully, as suddenly as the explosions began,

they ended. I surveyed the ward. Aside from broken windows and a few intravenous bottles, there was not any severe damage and no one was hurt. I then located the "combat" physician; he was curled in a ball under the nurses' station desk. Quietly he stood and walked off the ward. Two days later he transferred back to Saigon.

A month or so after that occurrence, I was on my way to the Red Cross building, which was about two miles of dusty road away from the 67th EVAC. It was located alongside the adjacent runway and was a favorite spot because it served ice cream cones, sundaes, and other treats.

Dusk was settling in when I started walking back to the 67th. Max, who was a warrant officer friend from Pittsburgh, offered me a ride back in his jeep. Gratefully I climbed in.

We had not gone far when we heard a loud explosion and felt the ground around us heave. Being the expertly trained and fearless military nurse that I was, I screamed and ducked to the floor of the jeep. Max threw me a rifle and a helmet and told me to keep watch and shoot if necessary.

I was, thanks to my upbringing, not afraid of guns, at least small hunting rifles with creek rats as targets. I had even ranked high in marksmanship during basic training. But the idea of cavorting around in an open jeep with a thirty pound gun, wearing a thirty pound helmet and flak jacket, was a little over the edge.

"Are you completely out of your mind?" I shrieked back.

Explosions sounded in the distance, but all I saw was the barrel of the gun, and my life passing rapidly before my eyes. I jumped out of the jeep as we approached the nurses' quarters and ran (as best I could while hugging the ground) to the bunker.

SIX

Celebrities

Entertainers often visited military installations in Southeast Asia, especially around the Christmas holiday. Bob Hope was probably the most noted and the most publicized, but others, with or without much publicity, came as well. Needless to say, these visits were greatly appreciated and anticipated. After Thanksgiving, the 67th EVAC personnel eagerly awaited news for possible celebrity entertainment, just as those in Saigon or Da Nang waited. Unfortunately, the 67th EVAC didn't make the entertainer cut.

We were therefore surprised when, one early December afternoon, a portly gentleman strolled into the medical ward. I immediately recognized him as Sebastian Cabot.

For those of you younger than fifty, Sebastian Cabot was an English actor. He was on a TV show in the '60s called *Family Affair.* He played the role of a butler to Brian Keith, the actor who played opposite Maureen O'Hara in *The Parent Trap* (original version).

Mr. Cabot was such a pleasant man, very friendly to all the patients and staff. He shook our hands and thanked us for our service to our country. What a boost his visit was for us. It felt so good to be appreciated.

A different encounter occurred a few days before Christmas. Not having anything else to do until I reported for work in a few hours, I walked over to the Red Cross building. A few other nurses and corpsmen were already there, so I joined them in a game of cards.

Surprisingly, I was actually ahead when I realized I had only an hour to get back to the hospital for duty. I ran out the door and slammed head first into a person who looked like King Kong, in combat fatigues and boots. I tilted up my chin to get a better look at Mr. Kong's face, and I stared in speechless amazement.

This gargantuan person was none other than Fess Parker. Fess starred in many popular TV shows and movies, including playing Davy Crockett and Daniel Boone. I watched one of his shows weekly when I was a kid.

The head-on collision must have caused brain damage, as well as the inability to speak, because I could not remember his name. So, as I stood there with my nose to his sternum, I said "Golly, you're Daniel Boone!"

He looked down at me and in a very deep voice said,

"Yep." Just like that! He didn't correct my error or look frustrated or anything; he just smiled.

I tend to talk a lot when I get nervous or excited, and this time was no exception. Words fell out of my mouth at such a rate that I'm sure Mr. Parker thought I was a lunatic.

As sudden as I started talking I stopped when I realized I was late for duty. I turned and started jogging down the road when he called out, "You want a ride to the hospital?"

Boy, did I ever.

You should have seen the looks on the nurses' faces when I showed up at work in a jeep driven by none other than Fess Parker. Their jaws dropped so much that their chins had road burns from hitting the pavement. They were so envious.

In Buddhist Vietnam the Christmas holiday took on a different image. The hot and rainy jungle replaced the cold and snow of home.

> — Elizabeth Norman, *Women at War:*
> *The Story of Fifty Military Nurses Who*
> *Served in Vietnam,* p. 24

SEVEN

Christmas in Vietnam

I loved Christmas, and still do. Nothing could deter me from celebrating, even without family. Seeing Sebastian Cabot and literally running into Daniel Boone, aka Fess Parker, just added to my resolve that we could have a beautiful Christmas. All we needed was a tree, some decorations, and presents.

Finding space for a tree was not a problem, because Cindy and I bunked in the laundry room, along with six other nurses.

Truthfully, it was not as bad as it sounds, because the room was large and attached to a former beauty shop. A shower stall was set up in the corner, and the attached beauty shop had sinks and hair-dryer chairs. However, the washers and dryers for the laundry had long since departed, which was good because otherwise there would not have been room for us to sleep.

Anyway, a few days before Christmas several of us headed out to look for a tree that we could chop down and put in our room. Realizing that a blue spruce or similar pine was not locally grown, we settled on a willowy kind of tree. It was of medium height and rather fluffy, and would look good once decorated. I don't remember how we got it chopped down or even how we managed to secure it in a pan of water, but we did.

We were all in great spirits as we scrounged paper, ribbons and anything that would serve as tree decorations. Our tree didn't have any lights, but that was not a problem. As necklaces and bracelets took their place among the branches and other decorations were added, our Christmas tree became a true sight to behold. Nurses, doctors, and corpsmen stopped by to admire our work of art.

As Christmas Eve approached, we were all anticipating packages from home. Very few had arrived so far, but we knew our presents were out there ... somewhere. Then we received the news; most of the packages from home had been stolen, or at least that was what we were told. Evidently thievery around Christmas was a routine problem. One would assume that the military could safeguard the soldiers' packages after a few years of having them stolen. But obviously that was not high on the priority list.

In the meantime, our chaplain was planning a special Christmas service. He "volunteered" several of us nurses to sing Christmas songs, and a corpsman volunteered to provide accompaniment on his guitar.

The night sky was clear and warm on Christmas Eve as we joined hands and sang hymns. It was a very solemn service that ended with most of us crying. We missed home so much. Thankfully, the night sky was also clear from mortars.

On Christmas morning those of us not on duty sat around the tree and gave each other presents that we had either made or bought at the PX. We later headed to the mess hall where Red Cross volunteers were giving ditty bags loaded with candy and needed toiletries.

Then, we stood in the mess line, anticipating a wonderful Christmas dinner equal to or better than that served at Thanksgiving, when we were served turkey, ham, potatoes, and all kinds of dessert.

Perhaps disappointment is part of military life, because the much expected wonderful dinner did not happen. We had the same grub as usual, served with lots of rice and bean sprouts. It was like any other day.

I guess it was time to get back to the war.

*The women adjusted to cold showers, latrines,
and small shared living quarters called
"hooches" in the army and air force and
"cabins" in the navy.*

> — Elizabeth Norman, *Women at War:
> The Story of Fifty Military Nurses Who
> Served in Vietnam,* p. 20

EIGHT

The Hooch

Cindy and I moved out of the laundry room and into our own hooch in early January. Just to clarify, during the Vietnam War era, hooch referred to a thatched hut, not moonshine or marijuana. Loosely speaking, any sleeping room was generally called a hooch by those serving in Southeast Asia and Thailand.

The women's compound at the 67th EVAC was a square, flat-topped wooden barracks structure surrounding a grassy courtyard. This barracks was divided into units which housed four women, mostly nurses with the occasional Red Cross worker.

Each unit was composed of a metal shower, toilet, and sink, flanked by two bedrooms large enough for a set of bunk beds and a small desk. There were no windows, but each bedroom area had a wall-unit air conditioner, which worked at least sixty percent of the time.

Cindy and I bought a little refrigerator and hotplate from the previous occupants and scrounged a small table that barely fit into our room and some blue paint. Blue footprints marching up the walls and across the ceiling served as wall art, as well as pictures of family taped to the walls.

Shower time was a challenge, especially if leg shaving was involved. First, there was no hot water, the metal stall was small, and there were insects — lots of insects.

Particularly distasteful were the roaches. One roach, whom we nicknamed George, was about five inches long and had one antenna shorter than the other, so he was easily identifiable. George was a frequent admirer during shower time, but always avoided the toilet area. My bunkmates and I were actually growing fond of him and no longer shrieked whenever he peered around the corner while we showered.

However, George's brazenness and lifespan reached its limit one night when Cindy found him snuggled under her pillow. By the time the death blows were over, there was nothing left of poor George to bury.

NINE

Daily Life

Life was often mundane at the 67th, except when being mortared.

Medical personnel worked twelve hours on duty, six to seven days a week, depending on the amount of combat activity and the number of casualties. A full work week was probably a good thing, because there was not a lot to do otherwise. The Military Assist Command Vietnam compound (MACV for short) was not far by bus. So going to the Post Exchange to shop for canned goods, electronics, and other non-clothing items was always an option during the day.

Occasionally a group of nurses and corpsmen would hop a bus to go to the beach. It was a convoluted trip on trail-like roads, but the beach and water were well worth the dust and bumps. The sand on the beach looked like fresh snow, stretching as far as you could see. And the water was a clear blue near the shore, and then purple farther out. There were shells of all sorts: large conch, starfish, and even cuttlefish backbones scattered in the soft sand. It was surreal to think that people were fighting and killing each other not far from where we stood.

An old-fashioned bathhouse, near the beach, was available for us to change into and out of our swimming suits. It was an open type of facility, no private stalls or anything similar. One afternoon, after spending time on the beach, I was in the bathhouse, naked, and starting to put on my fatigues when several Vietnamese women walked in. Circling me, like kids playing Ring Around the Rosy, they touched my hair, my breasts, and my clothes, all the while giggling and talking rapidly to one another. To me, because I did not understand their language, they sounded like magpies sitting on a fence.

While they circled, I just stood there, stuck to the floor. I didn't know what to do; should I act angry or just keep quiet. We had been indoctrinated during basic training to the Vietnamese culture (sort of), but I was not prepared for this type of inspection. I had no idea what they said, but I figured they were discussing how funny I looked, because of their laughter. I was a head taller than they, blonde, with light skin and green eyes. They were slightly built with dark eyes and long straight black hair. I was uncomfortable, not so much because of their scrutiny or anything they did, but more because I realized I was an uninvited stranger in their country, an invader, and had no right to be there. But I was there — whether they or I liked it or not.

Evenings off were usually spent either sleeping or in the Officers' Club, drinking. Games associated with drinking were the norm, and though these games varied from night to night, they usually ended the same: in drunkenness.

Talents in the alcoholic beverage drinking arena were particularly appreciated. One nurse had a unique flair for drinking flaming alcoholic concoctions. Perhaps it was because she had long red hair. How she did it, no one knew, but as she drank the fiery liquid, she would flip her long hair back, creating the illusion of Vesta, the Latin goddess of fire. It was a wonder to behold and quite frankly bruised many male egos as they failed in their attempts to best this fire-drinking, redheaded femme fatale.

Some evenings USO bands played at the Enlisted Men's Club or the Officers' Club. During these times, dancing was the main attraction and was enjoyed by all. It didn't matter if officers went to the enlisted club or enlisted men came to the officers' club.

There were also parties in the nurses' hooch, at least weekly. Usually everyone came, except those on duty. We really did party a lot, and we obviously drank a lot, but we worked hard a lot. Maybe it's not the same, but at the time it was.

If there is anything at [the] table that we don't like ... [we] shall take it thankfully, remembering Who had to ask a poor woman for a drink of water.

> — Florence Nightingale, *Florence Nightingale to Her Nurses: A Selection From Miss Nightingale's Addresses to Probationers and Nurses of the Nightingale School, St. Thomas's Hospital*, lines 608-9

TEN

Wham, Bam, Thank You, Spam

I was not much of a cook before going to war. My state-side specialties consisted of a half-decent spaghetti meat sauce (oregano was the secret ingredient), stuffed pork chops, and meatloaf. Oh, and tossed salad, to which I have been known to add even the kitchen sink. So it was not unreasonable for me to eat meals prepared by someone other than me. That was until I landed in South East Asia.

I never considered myself a cuisine prima donna. Growing up in rural America, I ate my fair share of corn meal mush (in liquid and fried form), rabbits, squirrel, and whatever came from the garden. Nursing school cafeteria food certainly had its bad points, but all of my previous eating experiences paled in comparison to Army food.

In basic training most of our meals, except dinner, were eaten in the Officers' Mess Hall, so the food wasn't too bad. But then came field exercises. I never thought ladles of food glopped together could be considered edible. Evidently the field cooks did. It seemed the higher the piles of whatever it was, the better.

And then just so we could have the whole wonderful Army eating experience, we got C-rations. It was then I realized how awful food really could be, and I couldn't imagine anything worse.

However, I imagined wrong, for in Vietnam horrible food took on a whole new meaning. I'm quite sure it wasn't the cooks' fault that the food was unidentifiable — most of the time. Truthfully, they had to cook something with what they had available. But, holy cow, it was bad.

Okay, to be fair, not everything was bad. There were certain meals, like spaghetti and pancakes, which were pretty good.

But the best was real eggs. The cooks knew how to flip those little white wonders to the perfect over-medium unmatched in the real world.

The down side was that real eggs didn't show up very often, so when they did the word spread so quickly that if you weren't in line early, you missed it. And, in that case, you had to suffer through the powdered eggs. As I mentioned previously, I was not a prima donna in the food department and could eat most things when hungry, but even I could not swallow powdered eggs.

Unless there was cheese. With cheese this powdered concoction became a wonder to the taste buds.

The cheese came via the always welcomed care package from home. Big blocks of cheddar were especially welcomed. The proud recipient of this treasured delight would carry his or her hunk of solid milk product to the breakfast chow line and stand there, smiling, with the cheese held forth like an offering to the food gods.

The cheese holder was revered — adored by all. Those already in the chow line would allow the holder to proceed to the head of the line. Then the cheese was gently handed over to the cook, who from long experience began the preparation.

Silently chards of this yellow delight were shredded into the goop of egg mixture, and the newly created omelet was served to the honored one. And, like a true god, the cheese holder shared with those in line this most precious gift.

Now there was the unspoken rule that if you were on poor terms with the cheese holder, you probably would not be a cheese omelet recipient. Therefore everyone tried to be pleasant to one another on mail day; especially when packages were delivered. One never knew if the person you yelled at earlier in the day would receive a cheese package. So it was the better part of prudence to keep bad feelings to yourself, at least most of the time.

And then there was the rice. There was always a thirty gallon drum of this white sticky stuff at every meal, even breakfast. I never ate rice growing up; Dad wouldn't allow it in the house. He said it was a WWII thing — even though he was on the European front, not the Pacific. But it didn't matter: no rice allowed.

In addition to the ever-present rice, there were bean sprouts; drums full of these uncooked, green stringy sprouts at the end of every chow line.

I had never before encountered a bean sprout, except, of course, in the ground ... growing up. And no self-respecting person in southwestern Pennsylvania would put a sprout of any sort into their mouth — willingly.

Particularly uncooked.

At that time in America, the only vegetables eaten raw were carrots, celery, tomatoes, radishes, onions, and lettuce. So I wasn't about to eat raw bean sprouts, especially in Vietnam. I may have been blond and naïve, but I wasn't stupid. I knew what was used for fertilizer in the fields in Vietnam, and it wasn't cow manure.

The monotony of mess hall meals was occasionally broken by the Koreans, who were mercenaries paid to fight against the Viet Cong. They were ruthless in battle but were good to have around, particularly when they brought steaks for our hospital staff. The post commander would order the patio grills made ready, instruct the cooks to bake potatoes, and then announce steaks over the PA system.

And, oh my, the steaks were so good: tender with

a flavor I can still taste. No one had the nerve to ask what animal these cuts of meat came from, and we really didn't care. For a brief moment in time, we drank and ate like real folks back home at a backyard barbecue.

Aside from the many, many things that we missed in Vietnam, the oddest seemed not celebrating normal U.S. holidays, such as Christmas, Hanukkah, Passover, and Easter, with special meals. With the exception of Thanksgiving, these religious days were treated much the same as any other day. I suppose it was because these holidays, except for Thanksgiving, were and still are Judeo-Christian celebrations, but it still seemed strange that our country, being "One nation, under God," could not at least provide something special to eat.

Anyway, much of the time I cooked my own meals — well at least supper. Cindy and I had a hotplate, and soon both of us became whizzes at boiling or frying delectable dishes.

There were a few hitches, though, to cooking: lack of cooking utensils, lack of storage, and lack of available things to cook.

Meat was the most scarce, at least the type of meat we would eat or were familiar with. But the one "meat" staple that was never scarce was Spam. The PX was loaded with shelves of this ham stuff. It was cheap and lasted forever.

With a little practice, I soon became the queen of

Spam. Did you know you could hash it, smash it, dice it, cover it with pineapple, fry it, put it in soups, and make a Spam salad out of it? Add little slices of precious hoarded cheese on top of saltine and you had appetizers. Slather it with mustard, slap it between two slices of white bread, and lunch was served. For supper, fry it in Crisco, add boxed macaroni and cheese, and chow down.

In war time, necessity really proved to be the mother of invention. And Spam brought out the culinary inventor in a lot of us.

ELEVEN

To Fraternize or Not to Fraternize

A week or so after New Year's, the commanding officer decided to re-enforce the non-fraternization rule. Enlisted personnel were strictly prohibited from the Officers' Club and vice versa. Not only that, but officers were prohibited from socializing with enlisted personnel, except for special company occasions. Enlisted men were also forbidden to enter the nurses' living quarters, including the central courtyard. Any infraction of this rule would result in the immediate transfer of the offending nurse to a field hospital near the DMZ (Demilitarized Zone). This was close to the border between North and South Vietnam, so it was not a good place to be.

Within the first week, we lost two nurses due to their ignoring the new rules, and a few more left in the ensuing weeks. It was eerie; one day a nurse was at work and the next day she was gone. No explanation from administration, just an empty hooch, and more work for the remaining nurses.

Ironically, the nurses had more in common with the corpsmen than with the physicians. Even though there were a few male nurses in the Army, the ones in our compound were all female. Most of the nurses and corpsmen had degrees, most were in their early twenties or thirties, and most were unmarried. On the other hand, the majority of male officers in the compound were physicians and most, if not all, were married.

This segregation irked me to the core. This was just not right. My little brother was enlisted, most of my cousins were enlisted, and the guys I worked with most were enlisted. It was as if the powers to be didn't care if nurses "fraternized" with married men, just as long as the men were officers.

Again my anti-authority character started to surface, in spite of my efforts to keep it under control. I wanted to do or say something about the stupidity of these rules, just to prove a point, but I also did not want to be transferred to the DMZ. Reluctantly, I decided the best course of action was to keep quiet — for now.

Then it happened. One afternoon, perhaps two months after the edict was delivered, I was sunning on one of the picnic tables in the courtyard of the nurses' compound. This was a large area with grass and several picnic tables. As I was catching rays, I heard voices in the compound area: female and male. Surprised, I looked and saw our chief nurse walking under the awning toward her hooch. Behind her, carrying several large packages, was a man, Sergeant Shaw. They didn't see me as they continued their way into her hooch and closed the door. The time had arrived for me to stand in the face of oppression.

I was working the night shift that week, so I asked one of the corpsmen from the medical ward to come over to the nurses' compound the next afternoon to catch some sun. He was well aware of the consequences of such an action and refused. After being accused of cowardice, he finally relented and met me at the picnic tables as planned. Just to make sure we would be noticed, I brought a radio and turned up the sound.

Nothing happened. No MPs swarmed down on me as we sat there talking. No announcements over the loudspeakers. Nothing. After about an hour he left, and I went back to my hooch, disappointed in my failed plan.

My disappointment didn't last long. The next morning, after work, I was given a message to report to the chief nurse at 1400 hours (2 p.m. civilian time). Instead of being excited at the opportunity to take a righteous stand, I was scared poopless with the reality that I would soon be packing and on my way to the DMZ.

I mulled over how to deal with my situation during the next six hours. It was clear that my one-woman crusade to end hundreds, if not thousands, of years of military rules was just plain idiotic. But I still needed a plan. As I walked to my appointment with death, I decided the best course of action was to act stupid and tell the truth, or at least as much of the truth as necessary. Then I would grovel.

The chief nurse was ready to see me when I arrived. Wearing my uniform properly and my best military face, I removed my hat and saluted. She did not invite me to sit or relax, so I stood there, cemented in place, trying to keep my knees from buckling. I was sure she could hear the loud hammering of my heart in my chest — I know I could.

"Do you know why you were summoned?" she said in her sternest voice.

"No," I replied.

"You were seen in the nurses' courtyard yesterday in the company of an enlisted man," she said. "Do you deny this charge?"

"No," I responded.

"Did you know this is an infraction of the rules?"

"Yes and no," I replied.

"What is that supposed to mean?" she demanded.

This was my moment of glory or defeat.

"Well, you see, ma'am, I knew enlisted men were not allowed in the nurses' compound or even courtyard. But two afternoons ago I saw Sergeant Shaw carrying packages and following you into your hooch. It's hard to keep up with restriction changes while working nights, but when I saw you and the sergeant together, I assumed the restrictions had been lifted."

Now came the groveling part.

"I sincerely apologize if I was in error, and I promise not to do this again."

As I glanced into her blue eyes, I knew I wasn't fooling her one bit.

She didn't flinch or even blink as she calmly said, "You should be sent to the DMZ, immediately."

I gasped inwardly. I was doomed.

Then she continued, "However, I will excuse this infraction once only."

"What? I'm not leaving? Did I hear right?"

Her stern voice broke into my silent celebration.

"Furthermore, Lieutenant," she barked, "from now on you will behave yourself. Do you understand me?"

"Yes, ma'am, I certainly do." I saluted and cautiously backed out her office door. If it wouldn't have appeared gauche, I would have bowed.

*And remember every nurse should be one
who is to be depended upon, in other words,
capable of being a "confidential" nurse. She
does not know how soon she may find herself
placed in such a situation; she must be no
gossip, no vain talker; she should never
answer questions about her sick except to
those who have a right to ask them; she
must, I need not say, be strictly sober
and honest.*

> — Florence Nightingale, *Notes on Nursing: What
> It Is, and What It Is Not*, lines 1461-1464

TWELVE

Coping

Coping with the everyday stresses associated with war was hard, if not impossible. Escape from reality became the favorite pastime not long after arriving in Vietnam. Aside from drinking alcohol, there was always talking about going home — to the real world: what our first meal would be, what movie we would see, what we would do, and so on. We anxiously awaited mail from stateside, goody bags from home, and catalogs from Sears, Roebuck & Co. It was amazing how a catalog connected us with real life and home.

Regrettably, escape from war sometimes took the form of contraband drugs. Marijuana was the most frequently used drug, but cocaine was a close second. Some days, if the weather conditions were agreeable, you could get high simply by walking through the picnic pavilion.

Other times you could see a hazy gray cloud hanging over a crowd of party attendees, like fog over London.

Most of the nurses preferred alcohol, because you did not get in trouble if you drank too much. Everyone understood and accepted the consequences of a hangover. However, illicit drug use was a different matter.

Sadly, one of the nurses who shared Cindy's and my four-bunk space succumbed to the use of drugs. We knew it and tried to caution her, but she would not listen. Probably we wouldn't listen if she tried to warn us about alcohol. But this was drugs. As her marijuana use evolved into cocaine use, her work deteriorated, and she became more and more isolated.

None of us could reach her. We wanted to talk with a supervisor, but there was no rehabilitation program in the Army and no excuse for drugs. Then one day she was gone; shipped out we were told. No reason given. Hopefully she received help.

A pastime soldiers have engaged in since the beginning of wars has been visiting local prostitutes, and the war in Vietnam was no exception. Many mornings I observed Vietnamese girls exiting the enlisted men's billet near the perimeter fence.

Of course, most of these visits included the transference of sexual diseases. So, once a week, any soldier or corpsman with a "drip" from his urinary apparatus would come to the medical ward for a shot of penicillin. Injection lines were usually long and completely without privacy. To make matters worse, the penicillin was thick, like cream, and so, in order to get it into a large enough muscle, it was delivered via a big long needle — into the buttock. Needless to say, this was a painful experience.

In spite of the pain there were a few soldiers that showed up in the penicillin line week after week. Repeated visits entitled the frequent flyer to receive the "corpsman special." Essentially, after the soldier dropped his drawers, the corpsman giving the injection would stab the point of the needle on a hard surface and then jab the blunted point into the soldier's behind.

The result was screams of pain, followed by lots of profanity, but unfortunately no decrease in extracurricular activities with the prostitutes.

Getting their field equipment was lots of fun. The girls received an olive drab herringbone work suit, consisting of blouse, well cut trousers, high field shoes, leggings, and helmet. They look at these garments dubiously.

— Helen Wells, *Cherry Ames, Army Nurse*, p. 131

THIRTEEN

Nursing in Combat Boots

Military nursing in South Vietnam was similar to stateside nursing, except for the occasional mortar attacks and the difference in the uniform. Rather than white uniforms, caps, hose, and shoes, we wore green fatigues, combat boots, and boonie hats. We also wore our dog tags, everywhere and all the time. The perfect Army nurse wore her baggy pants bloused (tucked into her boots), shirt buttoned neatly at the cuffs, and hair off her collar. Outside she always wore her boonie hat when in uniform.

Thankfully, most of us were not perfect. Sleeves were rolled up, pants were not bloused or tucked into our boots, because most of the nurses, including me, tailored their fatigue pants to fit snugly. Therefore, if they were tucked into boots, the look was just not fashionable. Also, hair allowed to be free-flowing was so much prettier than hair pulled into a ponytail, and the boonie hat just looked silly. Most of us believed that while we were in the Army and in a combat zone, we were still women, and we wanted to look as attractive as possible, even when wearing Army green and combat boots.

Another factor leading to a change in the nurses' working wardrobe was the method of washing clothes. The Vietnamese women hired by the military to wash clothes and bedding were unfamiliar with methods commonly used in the United States. They washed fatigues, underwear, sheets, and everything else in a large communal bucket. Considering that most of the nurses' panties were made of nylon, the heat and humidity associated with Southeast Asia, and the method of washing, it was no surprise that most of the nurses suffered from irritating vaginal infections.

Treatment for this affliction was not usually sought by the nurses, for several reasons. First of all, treatment was usually unsuccessful because of the constant exposure to the irritants. Also, most of the nurses were hesitant to be examined, because the medical people who performed the examinations were male co-workers.

The solution was simple: wear no underwear unless you were wearing a dress. However agreeable this remedy might be to some, I wasn't happy with the idea. First, I didn't know that most of the nurses wore no panties; it was never openly discussed.

More important to me was the recent arrival of my missing duffel bag and foot locker containing my underwear. The excitement of being able to wear my pretty undergarments versus male skivvies overshadowed the sage advice offered by my bunkmates, and so the infamous crotch rot set in after only a few washings. I was back to wearing skivvies or no underwear at all.

*"Symptoms of malarial fevers are (1st stage)
chilliness, shivering, face pale or livid, fingers
white ... (2nd stage) dry heat, skin burning
and flushed ... (3rd stage) profuse sweating."*

— Helen Wells, *Cherry Ames, Army Nurse*, p. 147

FOURTEEN

The 67th Evacuation Hospital

During the Vietnam War evacuation hospitals were set up to stabilize the seriously ill or wounded and then transport them to a larger facility for further treatment. Those not seriously wounded or ill were fixed up and sent back to combat. The usual stay at the 67th was a week or less.

Incoming patients during the triage process were assigned to either surgical or medical wards. Any patient who had, or could expect to have, surgery was housed in one of the surgical wards. Everyone else went to medical.

That's where I worked, the medical ward. Initially I was assigned to the surgical ward: neuro and orthopedic surgery. I was clueless. I was a pediatric nurse, for goodness' sake, and the patients were grown or nearly grown men. I looked at tubes and drains, and pins and bandages, and nearly threw up on a daily basis. After about a month of misery, the surgical head nurse had pity on me and recommended my transfer to the medical ward. I had no idea what this duty entailed, but I figured it had to be better than what I had been doing.

The medical ward was in a two-story wooden building at one end of the compound near the perimeter fence. Generally all health problems not surgery-related were cared for on medical. The first floor was the patient area, and the second floor housed the physicians.

The medical ward was shaped similar to the letter H. The patients' cots and the nurses' desk were contained in the outside structures, and the horizontal connecting structure housed the patient bathroom, showers, utility rooms and storage areas.

There were four exit doors on medical: one on each end of the vertical wards. I mention this because at least a third of our patients were there for psychiatric problems, and about a quarter to a third were there for drug-related issues: overdose and withdrawal mostly. The irony was that none of the doors on medical were locked, even the back doors, which were a few hundred feet from the perimeter fence. Obviously the powers that had organized the wards did not take into account the demographics of our military patient population in the '60s and '70s.

To illustrate my point, one day about mid-afternoon one of the corpsmen informed me that two of our patients were at the fence, probably engaging in a drug purchase.

While ordering the corpsman to notify the MPs, I high-tailed it to the fence to investigate. I watched these patients as they passed money through the fence to a little Vietnamese boy. In exchange for the money, I observed what I assumed was cocaine or marijuana being passed back.

Ordering the patients to halt, I informed them of their indiscretions and the jail time associated with such. I smugly watched as the MPs pulled up in their jeep, handcuffs in hand.

Unfortunately, these guys were smarter than I was, because at that moment they dropped their illegal stash by their bare feet, and in blue pajamas, with hands open and outstretched, they waited. The obviously illicit drugs littered the ground around us, but the patients were free to go back to the ward because the drugs were not on their persons. It was the patients' word against mine, and I lost.

Once again, I was utterly awestruck by the lack of intelligence within the military and wondered how we ever got this far in the war.

She would have to learn to strike just the right note with her soldier patients, not too familiar, and still with the warmth and understanding that was a big part of nursing.

— Helen Wells, *Cherry Ames, Army Nurse*, p. 13

FIFTEEN

Section 8 and Other Crazy Stuff

Similar to events seen in *MASH*, helicopters often delivered the severely injured to our hospital. The ill and less wounded soldiers were generally brought to the hospital in large groups and frequently in buses or ambulances from the field hospitals. There were always a high number of patients with malaria, hepatitis, drug overdose or withdrawal, and psychiatric cases on the transports.

Therefore, when notified of the imminent arrival of incoming patients, the medical ward staff prepared by organizing blood draws, cold showers for those with fevers, and restraints if needed. Usually these patients were brought directly to medical, saving the emergency room for triaging the wounded.

I was working the day shift when an unusually large number of injured patients were being brought to the hospital. While I was waiting for the onslaught of medical patients, one of my psychiatric patients approached me and asked, "What would you say if I told you I was going to slice my wrists?"

Being the expertly trained twenty-two-year-old psychiatric nurse that I was, and knowing that all sharp objects were under lock and key, I smugly responded, "Well, they're your wrists; do whatever you want." As I watched, my patient pulled a razor out of his pocket, sliced it across both his wrists, and darted out the unlocked ward doors trailing blood.

Horror washed over me as I yelled to one of the corpsmen to grab a Thorazine syringe and follow me. Running after my bleeding patient, I saw him enter the ER area where the newly arrived wounded were being triaged. Litters filled with injured soldiers covered the floor as nurses and physicians barked orders.

Chaos erupted when my patient grabbed a pair of bandage scissors from a nurse's pocket and started stabbing whomever he came into close proximity with. He jumped over stretchers, wildly stabbing, while I followed in his path with a loaded syringe. Thankfully, he used the blunt end of the scissors, so people were just angry, not hurt.

Over the cacophony of sounds, I heard a voice ordering me to control my patient. I turned toward the voice and saw that it belonged to the chief nurse, Lt. Col. Adams.

As I continued in pursuit, she followed, yelling nonstop along the way. A not-so-nice retort was about to burst out of my mouth when my corpsman leaped over a cot and tackled the wayward patient to the ground. I thrust the loaded syringe into his thigh, grabbed his legs while the corpsman secured his arms, and together we carted the soldier back to the ward, all the while listening to the ranting of Lt. Col. Adams.

Another memorable episode occurred early one evening. I was on duty when one of the medical patients, under psychiatric evaluation, was brought into the ward on a stretcher. He was covered in gravel, with scrapes and abrasions all over his face, chest, legs, and essentially the entire front of his body. His pajamas were torn at the knees, and his feet were bleeding.

According to the MPs accompanying him, this young soldier "took off" from the adjacent runway because he believed he was an airplane. So he asked if anyone wanted a flight back to the States. Receiving a negative reply, he climbed to the balcony at the airfield and "took off." Two days later he was air evacuated to Japan.

At times it seemed that lunacy ran rampant through the compound and was not limited to patients. Maybe it was a full moon, but one morning Lt. Col. Adams, the chief nurse, vanished. She had not been at breakfast, was not in her office, and did not answer the phone in her hooch.

A search of the hospital was unsuccessful. Finally,

a brave soul went to the nurses' quarters to investigate and found the chief nurse's door blocked to the top by a stack of sandbags. She was the only nurse with a phone in her hooch, but her line was found disconnected. She was there, in her hooch, unhurt, but mad as hell.

She was out for blood, and fortunately for the rest of us the perpetrators came forward and confessed. A few rather roguish physicians, with nothing better to do, had decided to have a little fun. Even though they were reprimanded by the commanding officer, the rest of us were totally awed by their heroic — if not stupid — deed.

R & R, short for Rest and Recuperation, always seemed to bring out the crazy in even the most serious of folks. Officers and enlisted personnel alike returned from their two-week excursions with wild stories that made the rest of us envious.

One story, however, was not envy-provoking. That story was about a short skinny nineteen-year-old corpsman from somewhere in Alabama. I don't know what his real name was, but everyone called him "Bloody."

Bloody was scheduled for R & R in Australia, a popular destination, especially for single male military personnel. Girls, drinking, dancing, and more girls beckoned many a man, and Bloody was no exception.

He also wanted a tattoo. Knowing he had to place his tattoo in an inconspicuous body location, he decided his chest was the best place, and being a true son of the

South, he decided a Rebel flag would be perfect.

Two weeks passed without Bloody getting a tattoo, and he was scheduled to return to Vietnam the next morning. So that last night, he got drunk — really drunk — and eventually passed out. He didn't regain partial consciousness until he was on the plane, and when he did he felt like his head would explode. He tried closing his eyes, but that didn't help. Bloody recognized that his pounding head was hangover-related, but that didn't explain the horrible, burning pain in his chest. Hesitantly, he lifted his shirt, took a peek at his chest and then just stared-open mouthed. His entire chest was one humongous, vividly colored Rebel flag — a bleeding Rebel flag.

"Oh s—t," he yelled. "When and how did this happen?" He tried to remember the previous night, but his mind wasn't cooperating. He questioned his fellow travelers, but no help there. All he could think about was how he was going to explain this to his commanding officer and his mother.

Boy, was he in trouble.

*"This is the Army! We want performance,
not excuses: An order is an order!"*

— Helen Wells, *Cherry Ames, Army Nurse*, p. 174

SIXTEEN

The General's Table

In late January 1971, Cindy and I were ordered to report to the commanding officer, who informed us that we had been chosen to represent the 67th EVAC Hospital at a dinner in Da Nang. Apparently the general of I Corps had mentioned to his aide one evening that he missed dining with American women, better known as "round eyes" in Southeast Asia.

Hoping to please his boss, this aide sent a message to all the hospitals within I Corps requesting each commanding officer to send two nurses for the purpose of granting the general's wish. The date was set, plans made, and orders given.

I should have been flattered, but I wasn't. I did not want to go. Several reasons came to mind, not the least of which was the fact that my oldest brother was arriving in

Vietnam around the same time as the planned dinner. I had not seen Gene for nearly two years, and I did not want to miss seeing him. We were short-staffed, and it was close to the anniversary of the Tet offensive. This usually meant an increase in casualties, and I hated leaving everyone in a bind. Finally, I could not fathom anything I would rather do less than being the female entertainment for some general, boss or no boss.

However, in the Army, if your commanding officer orders you to go to Da Nang to entertain a general, you go, especially if the order is followed by the threat of a court-martial if you refuse. And you would be happy about the trip and be nice. So Cindy and I located dresses, stockings, and dress shoes, packed our makeup, and set off for Da Nang.

We arrived early in the afternoon of the planned dinner and were greeted by an officer in charge of our well-being. We had a brief opportunity to look around and met many of the other female nurse invitees. We then dressed in our best borrowed outfits and joined our assigned escorts for the short drive to the general's mess hall.

The general's mess was a large ballroom type of hall. It was in the shape of the letter L. White tablecloths and napkins, crystal, and silver were set on round tables for parties of eight: four nurses and four male officers per table. Around the corner was the general's table. It was long and full of high-ranking officers. All the male officers were dressed in khakis, rather than fatigues, and the wait-ers, enlisted men, were dressed in white uniforms. There was music off to one corner, but I do not remember whether it was live or taped entertainment.

After drinks were served, the general stood and thanked us for coming to dinner. Then, after saying what a pleasant surprise it was to be surrounded by beautiful American women, he sat down. That was it.

Here we were, eating wonderful food, drinking excellent wine, and then dancing with our escorts at the officers' club, while back at the 67th, nurses were covering our backs. We left our hospitals short-staffed for three days at the most dangerous time of year so that an aide could impress his general.

The personal, positive side of this trip was being off duty for three days in a row. That never happened at the 67th. A fancy dinner and dancing afterward was really not that bad either. Another positive to this trip was while in Da Nang, I found a nursing school classmate who had also been my roommate during basic training. She was one of the first of our basic class sent to Vietnam and so was scheduled to go home in a few months. It was great seeing her.

The day following the dinner, all of us were invited to tour the hospital ship Hope. She was empty of most staff and all patients, as she was preparing to go out to sea during the anniversary of the Tet Offensive.

My, what a beautiful ship she was. All white: white floors, ceilings, beds, linens, and everything. This ship looked like an angel with unfurled wings resting on the azure-colored sea compared to the green caterpillar-like Army Evacuation hospitals spread out on the ground.

That evening ended after more drinking and dancing at the Officers' Club. Then it was time to leave, even though it seemed we had just arrived. As we left the next morning, I admitted, grudgingly to Cindy, that I was glad I came, even if it was under the threat of a court-martial.

However, my joy was short-lived after we arrived back at the 67th. The hospital had been swamped with casualties since we left, and everyone was exhausted. Fun time was over. It was time to get back to the war and the work of repairing wounded soldiers so that they could fight again.

SEVENTEEN

Remembering the Patients

Without the patients, soldiers, civilians, and innocent bystanders, there would be no story. Actually, they are the story, because they were the reason that I and probably all the nurses came to South Vietnam. Caring for those in need, both mentally and physically, was and continues to be intrinsic to the nursing philosophy: in times of peace and even more in times of war. The war in Vietnam was no exception.

For many years after the war ended, I refused to think about or dwell on the patients I nursed. I didn't want to remember — I wanted to put that part of my life as far from me as possible. Plus I took care of so many soldiers that remembering each and everyone would have been impossible.

Yet my mind sometimes traveled back to Vietnam

and to the people I nursed, and I wondered about them: how they had fared since I last saw them — forty years ago.

One of the soldiers that I remembered came to medical from the surgical ward. He had an orange-sized lymph gland on his neck, and he was very ill. The biopsy was negative for cancer, but what caused the gland to grow was a mystery.

In spite of antibiotics and other medications, his condition continued to deteriorate. He became delirious and started spitting at all of us, he was incontinent in his bowel and bladder, and then one night he started having seizures.

Grasping at straws, the doctor in charge of medical decided to repeat all the lab work, including a spinal tap. When all the specimens were collected, the physician took them to the lab and conducted his own analysis.

It was about 1 a.m. when the doctor called with the report: bubonic plague. No one could believe it. Bubonic plague was a disease from the Middle Ages — not the twentieth century. At first we were excited — what a discovery! And then we were afraid — bubonic plague was extremely contagious.

Out patient was immediately placed in isolation, and the appropriate antibiotics were started. Within twenty four hours he was awake, and by the end of the week he was stable enough to be transferred to Japan. We all celebrated his miraculous recovery.

What we did not celebrate was the injection of streptomycin that everyone who had come in contact with the patient received. Thankfully, none of the staff or other patients on the medical ward became infected.

Speaking of preventing the transmission of infectious diseases, the 67th EVAC had a unique method of isolating patients: it was called portable bed screens. Three or four of these screens would be placed around the bed of anyone with a contagious illness, for example, hepatitis or bubonic plague. Gloves were used, but only if working with really messy or nasty stuff. Masks were occasionally used for respiratory infections, but other than that hand-washing was sufficient.

Along with soldiers, we also took care of civilian wounded. There was one patient that I never forgot, even when I wanted to. He was an eight-year-old Vietnamese boy and was the first patient I took care of when I arrived at the 67th EVAC. I was working on the surgical wards at the time, and, because of my pediatric background, he was assigned to me. This little boy had been inadvertently shot in the chest by our military when his father held the boy in front of him as a shield. I could not fathom a father doing such a thing to his own son.

Like everyone else, I heard stories of American soldiers inviting Vietnamese children to come closer to get candy or something, only to be blown up by the explosives hidden on these same children. But to be face-to-face with such an atrocity was more than I wanted to experience.

This little boy was understandably afraid. He had been shot because of his father, had received reparative surgery, and then had awakened in an American hospital. People caring for him could not speak his language, and he could not understand theirs. At least his mother was allowed to remain by his bed.

The boy healed slowly, but he did heal, and eventually he left the hospital for home. As a parting gift, his mother gave me a gold ring. Just looking at the ring reminded me of not only this one child, but of all the children who have over the centuries been thrust into the horrors of a war and not knowing why.

Another patient-related story also involved a civilian: a young Vietnamese woman. I was working one night on the medical ward when the nurse from surgical asked if I would come over and check one of her patients, a female. This young woman had been shot by enemy fire and had been transported to the hospital for surgical treatment of her wounds.

According to the nurses in surgery and recovery room, she frequently grabbed her belly while moaning, "Mama-san, mama-san." Supposing that she was trying to tell them that she was pregnant, the nurses told her in their best soothing voices that she would be okay.

More than likely the young woman didn't understand what the nurses were saying or didn't believe them, because the belly-holding "mama-san" crying continued. She was soon moved to the surgical ward and the nurse, checking her surgical wounds, found the woman's belly swollen — just like a pregnancy. In fact, like a very advanced pregnancy.

That's when she called me. Not knowing how to deliver a baby, she figured that I was the closest thing to a labor-and-delivery nurse, because I took care of children.

That rationale made no sense at all, but I agreed to take a look. Putting on my best professional expression, I placed my hands on her swollen abdomen, to which she whimpered, "Mama-san, mama-san."

The hospital did not have a fetal stethoscope, and ultrasound had not been invented yet, so I listened with my regular stethoscope. No rapid baby-like heart sounds — only regular tummy growling. The next step, I figured, was to examine her vaginal area. Putting on sterile gloves, I took a peek — no head peeking back at me. That was good.

"One more thing. When was the last time she urinated?" I said to the nurse.

"Ummm, I don't know," she replied.

"Okay, let's check this lady's bladder."

I inserted a small catheter into the patient's urethra, and as the catheter entered her bladder, a miracle happened — her belly started getting flatter. As the fluid poured out through the tube, the young woman sighed in relief. The other nurse and I looked at each other in disbelief: it was not a baby at all — it was pee. I was so thankful that I didn't have to deliver a baby, and when the young woman grabbed my hand and smiled, I knew she was also thankful.

Aside from a few guys, the American soldiers who were patients at the 67th EVAC were absolutely wonderful. They were respectful and extremely appreciative of the nurses who cared for them. Even though they were only at the hospital for a short time, bonds were often formed. The nurses listened as the soldiers shared about their families, loved ones, and home. If they had pictures, they shared those also. Sometimes a nurse would write a letter home for the soldier, if he requested, and sometimes a soldier asked a nurse to read a letter from home.

But the one thing these soldiers didn't share was their war experiences, and the nurses didn't ask. It wasn't from a lack of caring or even a lack of interest on the nurses' part — it was more like hearing it would bring the war into the sanctity of the hospital.

The hospital was the one place that was as close to the "real world" as we could get: the ugliness of war was forgotten amidst the work of nursing, and the soldiers had a brief respite from the killing of war or seeing friends killed. And so, during the twelve hours of work or the few days as a patient, the nurses and soldiers could pretend that the war was somewhere other than where they were.

EIGHTEEN

Singing in the Band

I love to sing. Since I can remember, I sang: old songs, new songs, religious songs, and just about anything singable to anyone who would listen. If there was a stage, I was on it. I was not terrific, but what I lacked in talent I made up for in enthusiasm.

Around the latter part of December 1970, a group of corpsmen decided to put together a band. Surprisingly, the commanding officer granted approval for this enterprise, so the guys quickly garnered drums, guitars, microphones, and speakers. My roommate Cindy had a beautiful voice, and the band members asked her to sing. I do not remember why she declined, but I jumped at the chance. I attended rehearsals, and after a couple of sessions I was in the group.

We named our band Southern Comfort, I guess because that was a favorite adult beverage, and all the members, except me, were from the South. My contribution to the band, aside from wearing rather short skirts and singing a few songs, was to write down song lyrics. I spent hours in my hooch with headphones on, listening to songs played on my reel-to-reel tape player. I had them all: Diana Ross and the Supremes, the Temptations, Creedence Clearwater Revival, the Beatles, Bob Dylan, and many more.

Our band's first performance was scheduled for the Officer's Club at the 67th and the date was rapidly approaching. I wish I could report that I was ready and excited, but I can't because I wasn't. I was so apprehensive at the thought of standing in front of all those men, pretending like I was a singer, that being tied to a stake and set on fire had more appeal to me.

I looked over the crowd of cheering men and just knew that as soon as I opened my mouth I would get booed off the stage. I'm not a singer — I'm just pretending. So I did as any mature person would do: I belted down a couple of shots of bourbon. That helped a lot; probably too much, for by the end of the performance I was well on my way to oblivion. But I sang and I wasn't booed off stage.

After that, we performed several times at the Non-Commissioned Officers' (NCO) Club and once more at the Officers' Club. Then we received an invite to a club on a different post. It was a good performance, and we were well received. It took a while to pack the equipment in the truck and so it was late when we headed back to the 67th EVAC.

No sooner had we unloaded the truck than the earth erupted. Waves of heat, light, and sound rushed toward us like waves crashing on a beach during a storm. A shock wave, much like after an atomic bomb explosion, knocked us to the ground. Before the second explosion erupted, we found cover in the X-ray room, under the table.

Later, we discovered that the explosions were caused by enemy mortars hitting the nearby ammo dump. Thankfully, the mortars missed the hospital directly. The blasts caused structural damage only to several of the buildings, but no casualties, unless skinned knees, bruises, and soiled underwear counted.

As to the band, my career was short-lived. There were rumors that the USO was considering our group for the entertainment circuit, but this did not happen for several reasons. We were medical personnel and very much needed at the 67th. Also I was an officer and the other band members were enlisted, and because of the no-fraternization rule our choices for gigs were extremely limited.

With a sad heart I left the band. But it sure was fun while it lasted.

Cherry was inclined to plunge headlong into adventure and let courage take care of itself. It usually did. Maybe what she needed was less impulsiveness.

— Helen Wells, *Cherry Ames, Army Nurse,* p. 13

NINETEEN

The Air Force Dance

The Army throws a good party, but the Air Force throws a great party. North of the 67th EVAC was a small Air Force base at Pho Cat. It was situated, I think, in some mountains, or at least hilly terrain. USO bands, usually from Australia or Thailand, showed up occasionally to provide entertainment. The bands were terrific and always had at least two skimpily clad females singing and gyrating on stage.

The downside for the flyers was the lack of female dance partners, because nurses were not stationed at the smaller or outlying Air Force bases in Vietnam. So when a band was scheduled, the call went out to the nurses at the 67th. Those off duty were invited to attend, and quite a few did, even though leaving the compound was prohibited without permission, and permission was never granted. Of course, details like that never stopped nurses.

One Friday night, when I was off duty, the call came through. A band was playing that night at the base, and we were all invited.

I was ecstatic: my first Air Force dance. Getting there was no easy feat, however. Tucking our dresses into our fatigues and carrying shoes and makeup in our packs, we sneaked out the gate and into a nearby field. Within minutes a helicopter landed, and we climbed aboard.

After a short flight we arrived at the base and were surrounded by officers in flight suits. It was like being a princess in the fairy tale, "The Dancing Princesses," as we danced the night away.

As a friend once said, "It just doesn't get much better than this." And it didn't. We danced and drank and danced some more until early in the morning, and then the unthinkable happened — blaring sirens.

The pilots and crewmen were called out on a strike, and we were stuck without a ride back to the 67th. To complicate matters, several of us were scheduled to work that morning. If we didn't report to work we would be court-martialed, and if the commanding officer discovered where we were, we would likewise be court-martialed. The immediate future looked dismal.

Frantically we searched for a ride back to the 67th. A ground crewman finally located a pilot not on duty. Without hesitation he agreed, but he could not leave until 0700 hours, an hour after we were to report for duty. I did the only thing I knew to do: I called the head nurse of the medical unit and begged. Mercifully, she covered for me until I made it back. I am not certain what the other nurses did, but I am sure that groveling was involved.

*True nursing ignores infection, except to
prevent it. Cleanliness and fresh air from
open windows, with unremitting attention
to the patient, are the only defence a true
nurse either asks or needs. Wise and
humane management of the patient is
the best safeguard against infection.*

— Florence Nightingale, *Notes on Nursing: What
It Is, and What It Is Not*, lines 330-32

TWENTY

The Leprosarium

As I mentioned earlier in my story, my brother Gene was scheduled to arrive in Vietnam, and in January 1971 he did. It was great seeing him and catching up on all the family news. My little brother Jay left soon after I saw him and arrived home in time for Thanksgiving. So Mom and Dad had at least three of their four kids, including my older brother Larry, who was not in the military, home for the holidays.

Because Gene was an Army captain in the Quartermaster Corps and stationed at Tuy Hoa, not far from Qui Nhon, I was able to see him at least two to three times a month. On one of his visits to the 67th, we were invited to visit a leprosarium not too far from Qui Nhon. The invite came from Max, the warrant officer friend from Pittsburgh. I figured my commanding officer would not grant me permission to leave post, so I just left. I climbed into the back of the jeep and over cases of Coca-Cola, which Max said were a gift for someone Gene and I would meet later. Not a problem, unless we hit something or bounced hard enough to cause the bottles to break.

The jungle bordering the South China Sea provided a deep green canopy as we snaked our way to the leper colony. An hour or so later the dense jungle opened, and in the clearing by the sea stood a beautiful village.

A squatty nun, looking a lot like Sally Field in *The Flying Nun* television show, greeted us. I am not sure about her real name, but those who knew her called her Sister Coke because of her love for Coca-Cola. Therefore a trip to the leprosarium always involved bringing numerous cases of coke.

Sister Coke was absolutely delightful as she showed the three of us around the village. Beautiful ceramic tiles covered the cottages and all the structures. The open-air chapel was breathtaking in its blue and white tiled walls and floor.

According to Sister Coke, years before the Americans came to Vietnam, the inhabitants of the village were taught how to make tiles by the French nuns. Everyone had an assigned task, and over the years they created enough tiles to cover the outside of all the buildings in the village and the inside of the chapel. Even though afflicted with the terminal disease of leprosy, these villagers produced a beautiful, lasting memorial to the love of those who cared for them.

It was truly amazing to find everything so clean and fresh. A few of those infected by leprosy came out of their rooms to meet us, smiling broadly. However, most stayed hidden within the confines of their huts.

As we walked among the buildings, we noted quite a few tiles engraved with names of American servicemen who had been killed in the war. Sister Coke explained that American servicemen frequently visited the village and sent home pictures. Sadly, many of these men had been killed in combat. Their families wanted their sons, husbands, and fathers remembered, so they sent money for the tiles as a memorial.

As the afternoon grew toward evening, we climbed into the jeep for the ride back to the 67th. Visiting with Sister Coke and seeing the village was such a sobering experience that conversation was minimal. I am not sure what thoughts traveled in Max's and Gene's minds, but mine was filled with wonder and sadness — wonder at the propensity of the human spirit to create such beauty from the devastation of a deforming disease and sadness at the waste of human life from war.

Yet, popular novelists of recent days have invented ladies disappointed in love or fresh out of the drawing-room turning into the war-hospitals to find their wounded lovers, and when found, forthwith abandoning their sick-ward for their lover, as might be expected.

— Florence Nightingale, *Notes on Nursing: What It Is, and What It Is Not*, lines 1624-26

TWENTY ONE

Men, Sex, and Other Lies

The saddest part of being a female in Vietnam, or even in the military, was dealing with the underlying belief that women served in the armed forces to provide sexual favors to the servicemen. I overheard more than once the conversation with people saying that nurses came to Vietnam only to make money in exchange for sex.

In fact, according to these experts, several nurses made "lots" of money over and above their salary doing certain extracurricular activities. Red Cross volunteers, crudely referred to as Doughnut Dollies, bore the brunt of these rude remarks, more than the nurses did.

Perhaps there were females who profited from their unique status in South Vietnam, but that was not the norm. Most of the nurses came because of the altruistic belief that their duty as a nurse and an American was caring for their country's wounded. During their time off from the horrors of war, these nurses simply wanted to relax and have fun.

Perhaps the naïveté of the nurses impeded good judgment, because situations occasionally arose that caught them off guard. One particular ugly event occurred during an evening at the Officers' Club. Cindy and I, along with several other off-duty nurses, were drinking, dancing, and singing along with the taped music.

An Air Force captain was at the club that night and bought several rounds of drinks for all the nurses. We were having a great time — until it was time to leave. That's when this captain started making sexual advances: first to me and then to Cindy. When both of us refused, he became belligerent.

We hurriedly left and ran to our hooch. Moments later there was a pounding on our door. Cindy opened the door, and this "officer and gentleman" pushed her aside and barged in. He hit me when I attempted to help Cindy.

Our bunkmates were next door and arrived in time to prevent further injury. The three of us were able to push him out the door while the fourth ran for help. Needless to say, this guy was never again seen around the nurses' quarters or the Officers' Club.

I admit it — we were young and naïve. Quite a few of us came from backgrounds that provided little exposure to the wiles of the opposite sex. At times the attention was ego-boosting. It was great feeling attractive and wanted, but not so great when sex was expected or demanded. The good news was that as the weeks and months went by, we became more secure in accepting who we were and why we were in Vietnam.

From girls, we became women.

The veterans [nurses who had completed their tour and were going home] felt sadness and guilt at leaving. There would be no more parties and quiet talks with friends. Their group would scatter. Reunions back home were unlikely.

> — Elizabeth Norman, *Women at War: The Story of Fifty Military Nurses Who Served in Vietnam,* p. 111

TWENTY TWO

Going Home

It was now March 1971. Changes were happening in U.S. policy toward the war. Rumors ran rampant throughout the hospitals in I Corps that supporting American and Korean troops were to be replaced by regular Vietnamese soldiers. Most of us wondered how we would function and to what extent our safety would be compromised. We had heard such awful stories that I, for one, was truly worried.

My brother Gene shared similar concerns and on one of his visits informed me that I could apply for an early release from my Vietnam tour of duty. I had forgotten the armed services policy that two or more siblings could not be forced to serve simultaneously in a war zone. Even though Gene had a wife and baby at home, he was career Army and needed to complete the entire tour. I did not.

The application to request transfer from a war zone

was long and in depth. I think this was a psychological ploy to keep us from seeking early release, because after ten pages I considered burning the whole thing.

But I didn't. I wanted to go home. I was sick and tired of this war, the defeated looks of the patients I cared for, the utterly senseless rules, and most of all I was tired of our inability to make positive changes in the lives of the South Vietnamese people.

My mother also needed me. She had been diagnosed with cancer two years earlier, and although her surgery and subsequent radiation treatments were successful, the stress of three of her four children being in a war was taking a toll on her. She was not doing well emotionally, so I wanted to be as close as possible.

I was allowed three choices for reassignment, so I picked East Coast USA, West Coast USA, and Hawaii. However, when I turned in my application form to the clerk, I was informed that I had to fulfill my Pacific tour. I could keep Hawaii on the list, but not East or West Coast USA. I could choose Japan or Korea instead, but I wasn't having it. "Send it on as is," I instructed the clerk bravely while I gambled on my future.

Six or so weeks later I was in my hooch when I heard a knock on the door; it was Lt. Col. Adams, the chief nurse. "Good news," she said. "Your orders for transfer were approved." But before I could let out a decent "yahoo," she added with a smile, "You are being assigned to Fort Gordon, Georgia."

Okay, that was East Coast USA, which was good. From her expression, though, something told me that there was a downside to her smiling announcement.

My suspicions were confirmed when she blurted out, "And guess what? I am being assigned to Fort Gordon also. I should be there shortly after you."

I groaned and said to myself, "What did I ever do to deserve this?" Then I remembered the errors of my past: I guess it was time for payback.

As I called Gene with the "good" news, I started thinking about leaving Cindy behind. We had shared the same quarters for the past fourteen months in Washington, D. C., and Vietnam, and I couldn't help but feel guilty that I was leaving. She still had six more months to serve. We talked late into the night for many nights, and as my departure date drew nearer I knew I would probably never see her or the other nurses again.

The procedure for "processing" out of Vietnam was more involved than "processing" into the country. About five days before my actual departure, I took the bus to the main headquarters at MAC V. I presented my papers to the clerk, who told me there was a mistake in my orders. I had to finish my Pacific tour of duty before going back to the States.

"Check the orders," I pointed out. "They specifically state that I am going to Fort Gordon, Georgia."

Disgruntled, he signed the paperwork and sent me

to the next station. The same comments were repeated by all the clerks I encountered along the way and over and over again I directed their attention to the orders.

I was finally finished with the first part of the processing-out procedure and was happily walking across the compound at headquarters when a young soldier fresh from the boonies approached me.

Saluting, he said, "Ma'am, I will give you $500 for two hours tonight." I didn't appreciate the audacity of his request, but I was going home. Nothing was going to interfere with my joy. So, returning his salute, I retorted, "Soldier, I am short [meaning I was leaving country really soon] and there is not enough money in the world to make me stay one minute longer than I have to. But good luck in your endeavor."

By mid-May it was time to leave the 67th, and with hugs, tears, and more hugs I climbed aboard the plane for Da Nang. It only took one day to complete I Corps out-processing, and then I was on another plane heading south. Nothing could deter me now; I was on my journey home.

I was the only female in the camp of servicemen awaiting transport back to the States. I had an entire two-story barracks to myself, with my own guard at the door. Unfortunately, the bathroom was outside, so middle-of-the-night pottying was limited.

After being surrounded and hounded by men for the past six months, I was over the thrill. In fact, I wanted nothing more than to be treated as a person and an officer.

So a plan formed in my over-tired mind. I still wore the gold band given to me by the mother of the little boy I took care of right after I first arrived at the 67th. He was the one who was inadvertently shot by an American soldier. Normally I wore it on my right hand, but when I arrived at Cam Ranh Bay I decided it was best to appear to be married.

Slipping the band on my left ring finger, I pretended that my husband's name was Gene and that he was a captain and still in Nam. It worked. I was able to talk, play pool, and eat dinner without being hit on or harassed. I guess I had missed this part of survival training in basic.

Twice a day a roster of those assigned to the next troop transport plane was posted. If for some reason you missed your assigned flight (like being drunk), you had to start the process over. After three days my name was finally on the list to leave. Fearing I would oversleep and miss the early-morning flight, I stayed awake all night.

The first layover on our flight home was in Japan. I had not been there before and happily discovered that the Air Force terminal was loaded with stuff to buy and eat. I purchased all kinds of gifts for my family. After several hours, we boarded the plane and headed over the Pacific Ocean. Everything was perfect until a young enlisted man became sick and then sicker.

A physician was on the plane and was actually sitting not far from the sick soldier. After a brief check, he determined that the young man had taken a boatload of drugs. Then the physician found me and "strongly" requested that I move to the seat next to the drugged soldier so I could monitor his condition and keep him stable till we landed. I couldn't believe my luck. Here I was on my way home and still taking care of kids on drugs. I mean, why wasn't he happy to be going home? It was fine if he wanted to ruin his trip home, but he didn't have to ruin mine.

The young soldier and I made it in one piece to the air base near Seattle, but I was still perturbed. I glared out the window as all the men, including the physician, debarked the plane while I sat there babysitting a really stupid kid and waited for the ambulance. The MPs and an Air Force nurse arrived, and shortly thereafter I was relieved of my guardian duty.

As I stepped out the door of the plane, my thoughts swirled back to a similar, yet different, experience six months earlier when I first arrived in Vietnam. Instead of the heavy blackness of night, there was now sunshine and crisp air of the day. Instead of grim-faced soldiers with helmets and machine guns, there were now unarmed soldiers simply milling around the tarmac, conversing with each other.

I was home, and the war was over, at least for me. I had seen and experienced things that Cherry Ames never had, and perhaps not even Florence Nightingale. The longing I had for adventure was finally gone.

At least that's what I told myself.

EPILOGUE

And the Rest of the Story

The Pacific Northwest sky opened just far enough to allow the drizzling rain access through the pines to the road below. The bus traveling on this road was filled with newly returned military from South Vietnam, heading for the Seattle airport.

As the bus crept its way through the mist, the passengers looked through the grungy windows in silence. Each seemed to be lost in thoughts so private that conversation was internal, not external.

What will it be like when I get home? Will I still feel the same toward my girlfriend, wife, boyfriend, fiancé? Will she or he feel the same toward me? Have I changed so much that no one will really know me or understand what I experienced to cause the change? In the silence, I could read the faces of each soldier and knew their thoughts: anticipation mixed with trepidation.

We slowly stepped off the bus, gathered our meager belongings, and entered the civilian world in the airport. Faces of other travelers gaped at us like we were aliens. Contempt was evident on a few, pride on a few more, and indifference on the rest. Numerous pairs of eyes watched as we headed toward the ticket counter, while surprise registered at seeing a military-dressed woman traveling with the soldiers.

The airport was gigantic, at least by my standards. I was lost — literally. I had no clue as to the method of obtaining a plane ticket in the military. My frantic expression must have been written in bold letters on my forehead, because a top sergeant approached me, saluted and said, "Ma'am, may I assist you in getting a plane ticket home?"

I wanted to hug him, and probably would have except for the protocol thing. Instead I returned his salute and simply replied, "Yes, Sergeant. I would be most appreciative." I hastily added, "I am going to Pittsburgh."

"So am I," he responded, and with that he smartly about-faced and marched toward the ticket counter.

"Ma'am?" I grumbled under my breath. "He must be as old as my dad and he's calling me ma'am! I will never get used to this darn military protocol."

A strong urge to use the ladies' facilities interrupted any further thoughts of the absurdity of military rules. I hurried to the nearest lavatory, and after relieving myself, looked in the mirror. The face reflected back was that of a stranger, or at least someone in desperate need of cleaning. I was unkempt, my clothes were wrinkled, my hair a disaster, and I had smeared makeup all over my face. I also had smelly pits. UGH!

I stripped down to my slip, and using paper towels and hand soap I started scrubbing myself where I could easily reach without too much exposure. Ladies in need of washing only their hands stared at me with questioning faces, but I didn't care. The water was hot and plentiful. I did what I could with my hair, put my uniform back on, and headed out to the terminal.

I soon located the sergeant. "Good news," he proclaimed. "We leave for Chicago in one hour, and we will arrive there at ten tonight."

I stared at him in amazement; I was really going home.

"But," he quickly interjected, "we have an eleven-hour layover in Chicago before leaving tomorrow for Pittsburgh."

I groaned.

Just then a thought occurred to me. My aunt lived near O'Hare Airport. So I placed a collect call to her and before I could ask anything, she said, "I will be there when you arrive. Then you will come to my home for the night."

True to her word, Aunt Betty met me as we deplaned at O'Hare. Hugs and kisses later, she whisked me to her home. Then she called my mom. After talking briefly, my aunt asked me what I wanted: a hot meal, sleep, anything.

I told her all I really wanted was a tub bath with lots of hot water and hair washing. This was not an easy request to make, for my aunt's basic premise was that two inches of water in a tub was more than enough for any normal human being to get clean. Any more than that was wasting water.

Therefore I was pleasantly shocked when Aunt Betty, without disparaging remarks, filled the tub to the brim, added bubbles, and told me to enjoy.

And I did. After at least four hours of soaking, I relinquished the tub. Although pruned in appearance, I felt wonderful.

Scrubbed clean and with hair fixed, I met the sergeant and the others heading for Pittsburgh at the airport later that morning.

"Damn, Ma'am," he exclaimed audibly, forgetting his salute. "You sure do clean up nicely."

Entering the huge aircraft bound for Pittsburgh, I was astonished when the stewardess took us to our seats.

"First class? This must be a mistake," I whispered to the top sergeant.

"No, Ma'am," he responded back to me. "Seems like you being a woman and back from the war softened someone's heart."

What a treat! The flight in first class was wonderful.

I think we were given champagne and a steak for breakfast, but perhaps I imagined that. I had not really slept for over forty eight hours, so maybe hallucinations were setting in.

I immediately spotted Mom and Dad among those waiting for the other passengers as our plane taxied up to the gate. They smiled broadly and waved as I stepped out of the plane and descended the steps into their waiting arms.

My folks looked absolutely wonderful and Pennsylvania never looked this great before. It might be rural and boring, but I felt like Dorothy in *The Wizard of Oz* when she said, "There's no place like home."

Author's Notes

You, the reader, may ask, "Why now? Why write a book about your Vietnam experiences forty years later?"

The answer is simple: it was time. Yes, the facts are probably distorted by the memories, but isn't that always true when telling a story?

Over the years, I have listened to a lot of men tell their war stories, and I am sure their stories were mostly true, with a little embellishment added; what was and what might have been.

There is nothing wrong with that. All of us choose to remember what seemed important at the time and forget what wasn't or what was too unpleasant.

And, as my veteran husband always said, "Why

mess up a good story with a few facts?"

As for me, I just wanted to tell my story in my words to my grandchildren and my great-grandchildren. I wanted them to know that their grandmother actually wore combat boots. Until the last two decades, women did not have an active combat-zone role, except as nurses and clerks. But we served. We didn't suffer the same, but we suffered. Our wounds may not show on the outside, but they are there nonetheless.

Military nurses have stories to tell, if given the chance. This story was my chance, in my own weird way. My intent was not to make light of the many horrors encountered by nurses in South Vietnam or to leave the impression that this war was fun and games for me. Rather, my intent was to demonstrate the absurdities of the war that I experienced.

The term "round eyes" comes from military slang used by American soldiers stationed in South Vietnam. In theory, anyone not Asian could have been referred to as "round eyes." In reality, the term was a little more sexist, and used to differentiate Asian women from non-Asian women.

The stories I told are true, at least to the extent of my memory. However, the names of most of the people in my story have been changed. Not that I think they would be embarrassed or offended, but to protect their privacy.

Those of you who were in Vietnam or are history

buffs will note that I did not identify the bases in Vietnam where I in-processed and out-processed. Since completing this story, I discovered from other sources that in-country processing for nurses was at Long Binh and processing out of Vietnam was at Cam Ranh Bay. I hope you will forgive me these omissions.